Oil Pulling Therapy The Beginner's Guide

How Oil Pulling Can Detoxify, Heal & Transform Your Body

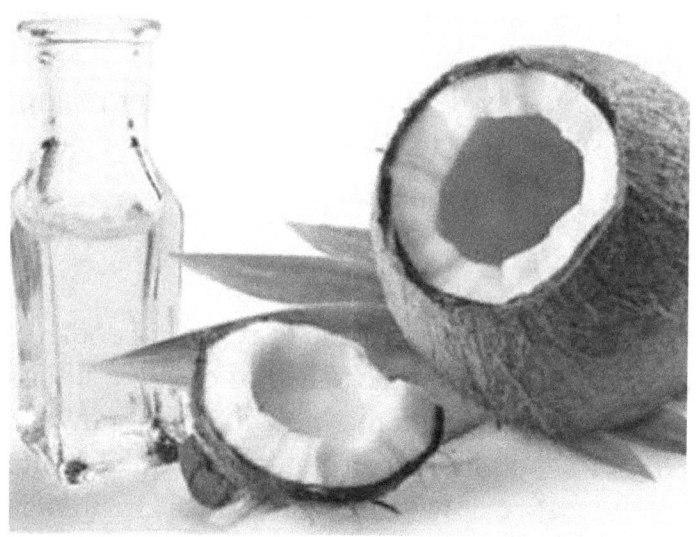

Copyright©2014 By Dr Brad Turner

Disclaimer

This book is intended to be a general guide, to raise awareness, and to help people make informed decisions in the context of their own personal circumstance.

As everybody's circumstances are different, so are the remedies you should seek. While many of the remedies in this book can be applied by almost anybody regardless of their conditions, they are not intended to and should not be relied upon to replace personal medical advice.

The author accepts no responsibility for any loss, be it personal or financial, as a result of the use or misuse of the information in this book.

If you have any doubts or concerns after reading this book, please speak to a doctor or other qualified person before taking any actions.

From The Author

Thank you for taking the time to read this book. As an author, I understand the importance of creating books which my readers will find both enjoyable and informative. If you have the time and feel generous, please don't hesitate to leave an honest review of this book.........Dr Brad Turner.

Contents

Introduction

Over the years, researchers have spent their time and effort studying the causes of diseases in the human body. Various equipment to enhance research have been developed, the first one being the microscope which was invented by Antoine van Leeuwenhoek in the late 1660's. This proved to be a major tool that enabled the modern man to know the existence of small single celled organisms. After keen studies, there was the realization that some of the single-celled organisms were useful, yet others were disease-causing. The mouth is a major opening into the physiological systems of humans, and this has posed a threat to the health of many humans, because micro-organisms use it as a gateway to come internally and mutually or parasitically feed on us.

In Ancient medicine, there is concrete evidence which suggests that our forefathers used oral hygiene as the number one remedy to stay away from diseases. So, how did they do it? There was the use of a simple idea, that suggested that if the mouth was the passage which connected the internal body to the outside world, then it's the main cause of many internal diseases. This keenly led to the research of herbal natural medicine that would cure all problems of the mouth and keep it healthy. The most famous way of doing it was the use of oil pulling.

Objectives of This Book
The objectives of this book were purely directed to every individual who would want to know the theories of oil

pulling. Some of the major aims are:

- To enable a person to know what oil pulling really means and some of its significance in early medicine.

- To describe some of the research that has been conducted to sideline the mythical and scientific aspects that concern oil pulling.

- To bring about the knowledge of how oil pulling should be conducted and some oils that should be used.

What is Oil Pulling?

Oil pulling is an ancient Ayurvedic remedy for oral health and detoxification. It involves the use of pure oils as agents for pulling harmful bacteria, fungus and other micro-organisms out of the mouth, teeth, gums and even the throat. It is also referred to by another name: Oil swishing. Its practitioners claim that it is not only capable of improving oral health, but systemic health as well, including a benefit in conditions such as headaches, migraines, diabetes mellitus, asthma, acne, and staining of the teeth. Its promoters claim it works by pulling out toxic accumulation, known as Ama in Ayurvedic medicine, and thereby reducing inflammatory effects. Oil pulling is one of the least studied wonders of science; in one study, sesame oil was found to be efficient in fighting plaque and the bacterial load in the mouth, however the scientist who conducted the experiment made an interesting analysis that it was less effective than chlorhexidine (a chemical mouthwash).

Is Oil Pulling Real or a Myth?

Oil pulling is real according to researchers and people who have had experience with it; however, there are some myths and misconceptions that come with it as well.

Realism of Oil Pulling

Oil pulling is considered realistic due to the following effects that come into play after using it:

- No or Lessened Sensitivity in the Teeth.

There are many men and women who have claimed that they stopped having undue sensitivity in their teeth immediately after gargling oil for a specific time, say 20 minutes. They continue to say that if after some time they stop their new habitual ways of oil pulling, the sensitivity usually comes back.

- Scientifically Proven.

Although no major experiments have been done to prove whether oil pulling really does work, there are some minor experiments and experimental ideas which included surveys that have been conducted to conclude that oil swishing is real.

- Evidence of Ancient Usage

There is hard evidence that shows that the Indians from ancient times were using oil pulling. In their traditional Ayurveda, which was an ancient Indian practice, gargling treatments such as "Kavala Graha" and "Gundusha" were used in the treatment of various bodily humors.

The above are but a few pieces of evidence that have shown that oil pulling was and is a reliable practice in the cure of many health problems within the body of humans and various animals as well. Despite this, there is also the elemental part that describes oil pulling as a mythical analysis. The evidence brought forth is such as that below:

- Lack of Totality in Experimentation.

   Majority of people would say that since there is no widely covered experimentation evidence, then there is a high possibility that the evidence brought forth to support its effectiveness could be vague and unrealistic. Some people, especially psychologists, have criticized the remedies that oil pulling claims by stating that the results may have occurred because the patients chose to believe they had been cured after using oil. "It is psychological", they said.

   This claim shows that there is not enough evidence to differentiate between realism and myths in oil pulling; however, time will tell after the effects are much greater. Although at the present time, the realism of oil pulling seems to be gaining the upper hand, especially in herbal medicine.

Scientific Research

At the 87th general session of International Association for Dental Research, scientists there reported on new studies that showed the relationship between oral and systemic diseases. They stated that it was something of a recurring theme between gum disease, infant maturity, stroke, and diabetes. The mouth is known to be rife with germs, harboring vast quantities of them. This is might turn out to be a very serious condition if proper oral hygiene is not observed. Despite this, there is also the natural way of dealing with oral bacteria: The efficiency of saliva. Our saliva contains enzymes that are able to break down many oral bacteria, hence keeping us safe from diseases. However, there are some germs and viruses such as polio virus, which may be uncontrollable and may cause gum infection. Most of the major internal diseases first are attracted through the mouth, and after some time, they then appear visible through the mouth. Some of the notable diseases include common cold, HSV (Herpes Simplex Virus), and AIDS among many more.

Some of the Scientific Studies on Sesame Oil and Oil Pulling

Sesame oil is especially high in the antioxidants sesamol, sesamin, and sesamolin.
It likewise holds a high amassing of vitamin E and

polyunsaturated unsaturated fats. These cancer prevention agents have been found to stop the assimilation of negative types of cholesterol in the liver. Different experimental studies have indicated the antibacterial limits of sesame oil pulling in the avoidance of dental depressions and gingivitis.

A study done in 2007 investigated the impact of oil pulling (with sunflower oil) on plaque and gingivitis on delicate and hard oral tissues. The results found that following 45 days of oil pulling, subjects indicated a factually critical decrease in gingivitis.

A late study, directed in the year 2008, found a striking lessening in the aggregate amount of microscopic organisms in the mouth and a general diminishing in dental cavities. The antibacterial action of sesame oil was additionally concentrated on and found to have an impact in the streptococcus mutans in the mouth.

Indeed, these studies demonstrated a general decrease of microscopic organisms from 10 to 33.4% in members, and following 40 days of oil pulling, members were found to show 20% in normal admonishment in oral microbes. A large portion of all members for this situation study demonstrated an intense lessening in weakness to dental transporters.

Testimonials

Beckinsale, a Chicago region blogger, used to gargle the oil in her mouth once a day. She now guarantees that her teeth look somewhat white around day five of oil pulling, and the

Eczema on her left foot started to clear up. From that point forward she has been proposing the same for her loved ones, and there have been astounding results. This has started an enthusiasm toward oil pulling in Chicago and her environs.

Should You Oil Pull?

Yes, and of course, everyone should oil pull, even those who do not accept and believe in its wonders. It is far better to try something once in a lifetime so that you can be sure if its effects are real or just mimics. If the effects are useful to you, then go ahead and embrace the product; however, if the effects are damaging, it is far wiser to let it be. The exception of who should oil pull only belongs to children below the age of five years, who haven't mastered the art of gargling. You should only oil pull by following the below guidelines to ensure that what you are doing is correct.

- Ensure the Use of Recommended Oil

   Not all oils can be used for oil swishing; there are those that have been tested and proven. It is usually better to do a lot of research on which oils to use when you are a beginner in oil pulling. Some oils aren't even used at all, such as petroleum oil which can cause physiological malfunctioning if ingested. The most commonly used oil for oil pulling is coconut.

- Seek Advice From an Expert or Someone With Experience

  Looking for advice is a very good idea, especially when the person giving the advice is mature enough in the field, that is to say, he or she has a lot of experience regarding the use of Ayurvedic remedies. It is usually much safer to have such a person around.

- Consistency

  When you start to oil pull, there is usually a need to be consistent; this is because most people, after finding the solutions to their oral problems, tend not to continue with the medication. This has resulted in recurrence of their problems which will prove difficult in treating. This is just one of the greatest side effects of oil gargling. Despite this, there might be the use of a different oil to regain your health.

- Amount of Use

  Despite the fact that a majority of the oils used for this purpose are almost considered as food, there is a required amount that a person has to take. If the maximum limit is reached and there is continuous usage, then there can be some damaging effect to the teeth or oral cavities. For example, they can dissolve the enamel and cement parts of a tooth to make it weak. Hence, if the required oil usage is once per day, then it should be kept at that.

Chapter 2

How to Oil Pull

The best and most basic strategy for pulling oil is carried out by putting around a tablespoon of icy pressed sesame oil into the mouth and gargling it for about 10-15 minutes, then spitting it out.

Different sorts of oil, for example additional virgin frosty pressed coconut, olive and sunflower have been utilized, yet sesame is viewed as the best. It is best to utilize exchange oils each time within request to experience the full benefit. This system for oil puling has multiple effects.

What Happens in the Mouth During Oil Pulling?

At the point when the oil is taken into the mouth, it first blends with the saliva transforming into a meager white fluid. Poisons from the saliva are then hauled out by lipids in the oil.

As the oil gargles in the mouth, teeth, gums and tongue, it keeps on engrossing poisons, normally finishing up turning thick, gooey and white. When this consistency is reached, it is released by spitting before the poisons are reabsorbed.

Oils to Use For Oil Pulling

There are many oils around; however, not all are used for this purpose. This is due to the fact that some oils are harmful to human physiological systems. Hence, there are recommended oils that are known for oil pulling. Also, there is a required maximum measure of the total amount that can be used in a given period of time.

Sunflower Oil

A non-volatile oil, which is extracted from sunflower seeds by the use of a mortar and pestle. Although there are versions of it that are industrialized, the pure natural sunflower oil is better for usage when it comes to oil pulling.

Other Uses of Sunflower Oil

- Used in the lowering of LDL (Low Density Lipoprotein) and prevents constipation

- Sunflower oil contains fatty acids which are essential during the Cori cycle

- Used in moisturizing the skin also, it has some use in the prevention of arthritis and the stimulation of wound healing

Side Effects of Sunflower Oil

- Contains a lot of essential fatty acids which may be harmful to the physiological systems of the body

- May cause allergic reactions in people who are sensitive to the Asteraceae/Compositae plant family. This family consists of members such as ragweed, marigolds, chrysanthemums, and daisies, among others

- Due to the large amounts of fatty acids found in sunflower oil, there is a huge risk of developing diabetes and also hardening of the arteries (Arteriosclerosis) , which may lead to death.

Another well-known oil used in oil pulling is the famous African nut called the *Coconut*. The nut has a variety of uses, some of which I have listed below:

- Used in the making of soap and lighting fires

- Used as a cooking oil

- Applied on skin and hair to make it soft

There are other oils that are associated with the healing power of oil pulling; however, they are not as effective as those mentioned above. Such kinds of oils include sesame, peanut, almond, and olive oils among others.

The Do's and Don'ts of oil pulling

Despite the efforts that Oil pulling has put up, there is a specific code and pattern that it must follow. These are the simple logical rules of do's and don'ts.

The Do's

When engaging in oil pulling, below are some of the things that must be put into action:

- Always ensure that you consistently use the required amount of oil pulling and that you do accommodate your oil pulling activity every day; let it be part of you in daily chores that must be done.

- Always spit contents into the garbage. This is a proper measure to ensure that hygiene is maintained at higher levels and standards.

- Try to educate others about the benefits of using oil pulling; persuade them that it's better to try out and realize the realities and misconceptions of it for themselves instead of waiting on others to tell them.

- Ensure that oils used for oil pulling are kept out of the reach of children since, if by any chance they swallow them, they can have some physiological difficulty

- Always rinse your mouth with clean water to ensure that all the contents of the oils have been removed from the oral cavity. This acts as a safety precaution to ensure that no oil deposits remain, since long exposure to oils that are used for pulling can damage the teeth.

- Always ensure that you buy the specified oil with government quality mark brand. Some oils are not up to standards.

The Don'ts

The don'ts that apply when doing Oil pulling are the most sensitive kind in its nature. If they are not taken seriously into consideration, the outcome can be lethal and damaging to yourself and those that surround you. Some of the MUST not do's when engaging in oil pulling are:

- You must never ever try to mix two different oils that are used in oil pulling; for example, mixing sunflower and coconut oils and using them at the same time. This can be lethal, since the two can form an entirely different substance that may end up harming its user.

- Never try to give oils to children who are below the age of five. This is because a majority of them will end up swallowing the constituents. This may be harmful since the amount of essential fatty acids ingested is not known.

- Do not ignore going to the dentist, for the simple reason that you are using oil pulling. This is because it has not been fully scientifically proven yet. To be on the safe side, it is usually safer to visit the doctor more often.

- Never forget to read the instructions and directions manual before using any kind of oil.

- Do not put oils near a fire, because this can lead to a very lethal case of a fire accident, since oils are flammable.

Mechanism of Oil Pulling

Oil pulling has a unique way of how it performs its effect on the human body. Researchers who have learnt its ways and mode of operation have come up with various experiments that would prove the reality of oil pulling and perfect treatment. Below is a demonstration of how oil pulling works.

Aim

The aim of the practice was to find out if saponification really does occur during oil pulling.

Materials used

-Lignans Bacteria

-Sesame

-Biuret and Beaker

Method Applied

Antibacterial activity in lignans and sesame oil were tested in a minimum inhibitory concentration of agar in both dilution and diffusion methods respectively. Saponification was done using titration of sodium hydroxide against fatty acid in the sesame oil. Swishing was done to finalize the procedure.

Observation

When the swished oil was observed under a light microscope there were deposits of micro-organisms, oral debris, and foreign bodies.

Results

Sesame did not have any effects on Streptococcus mitis, Streptococcus viridans and Streptococcus mutans. Oil pulling occurs during emulsification of sesame, and with increase of sodium hydroxide in titration, there is a definite indication of the possible saponification process.

The above clearly shows that oil pulling therapy is not just a placebo, since emulsification and saponification were clearly defined in the practice.

Chapter 3

What are the Benefits of Oil Pulling?

Various exploratory efforts done in the past show that oil pulling, particularly with sesame oil, can help general oral well-being. Particular utilization of sesame oil as an oral well-being executor serves to decrease the measure of S. mutans (germs) in both the mouth salivation and teeth plaque. It is accepted by researchers that the lipids in the oil haul out the micro-organisms as well as prevent the bacteria from adhering to the dividers of the oral cavity.

Also, oil pulling expands saponification in the mouth, making a foamy environment that washes down the mouth as vegetable fat is an emulsifier by nature. It is intriguing how the oil can rinse out hurtful micro-organisms and additionally lessen abundance of specific micro-organisms, by retarding growth.

The oils additionally help in cell rebuilding, and are identified with proper working of the lymph hubs and other inner organs.

Other Possible Benefits of Oil Pulling

They include:

- Overall strengthening of the teeth, gums, and jaws.

- Possible holistic treatment from TMJ and general soreness in the jaw area.

- Prevention of dryness of the lips, mouth and throat.

- Potential holistic remedies for gums that bleed.

- Prevention of bad breath from the mouth.

- Whitening of teeth.

- Prevention of diseases of the gums and jaws.

Gingivitis and Periodontal Diseases

Gingivitis, generally also called gum disease or periodontal malady, starts with bacterial development in your mouth and may end - if not legitimately treated - with tooth misfortune because of obliteration of the tissue that encompasses your teeth.

Difference Between Gingivitis and Periodontitis
Gingivitis (gum aggravation) normally goes before periodontitis (gum infection). Notwithstanding, it is paramount to realize that not all gingivitis advances to periodontitis. In the early phase of gingivitis, micro-organisms in plaque develop, causing the gums to get aggravated and to effectively drain throughout tooth brushing. Despite the fact that the gums may be chafed, the teeth are still immovably planted in their attachments. No irreversible bone or other tissue damage has happened at this stage.

At the point when gingivitis is left untreated, it can development to periodontitis. In an individual with periodontitis, the internal layer of the gum and bone force far from the teeth and structure pockets. These little spaces between teeth and gums gather garbage and can get tainted. The body's immune system battles the micro-organisms as the plaque spreads and develops underneath the gum line. Poisons or toxins - handled by the micro-organisms in plaque and the body's "great" chemicals included in battling diseases - begin to break down the bone and connective tissue that hold teeth set up. As the ailment advances, the pockets extend and more gum tissue and bone are wrecked. At the point when this happens, teeth are no longer tied down, they get detached, and tooth misfortune happens. Gum disease is the leading reason for tooth misfortune in grown-ups.

Reasons for gum ailment

Plaque is the essential driver of gum malady. Then again, different elements can help periodontal malady. These include: Hormonal progressions - for example, those happening throughout pregnancy, adolescence, menopause, and month to month period - make gums more touchy, which makes it simpler for gingivitis to create. Ailments may influence the state of your gums. This incorporates ailments; for example, disease or HIV that meddle with the resistant framework. Since diabetes influences the body's capacity to utilize glucose, patients with this disease are at higher danger of creating other diseases, including periodontal sickness and pits.

Medication can influence oral health, on the grounds that some reduce the stream of salivation, which has a defensive impact on teeth and gums. A few medications, for example the opposition to convulsant prescription Dilantin and the anti-angina drugs Procardia and Adalat, can result in irregular development of gum tissue. Unfortunate propensities – smoking, for example - make it harder for gum tissue to repair itself. Poor oral cleanliness propensities, for example not brushing and flossing consistently, make it easier for gingivitis to create. A family history of dental maladies could be a helping component for the advancement of gingivitis. What are the side effects of gum illness? Gum illness may advance easily, showing few evident signs, even in the late phases of the malady.

Despite the fact that the side effects of periodontal infection frequently are unobtrusive, the condition is not by any stretch of the imagination without cautioning signs. Certain side effects may indicate some manifestation of the malady. The side effects of gum malady include: Gums that drain throughout and after tooth brushing, red, swollen, or delicate gums, tenacious awful breath or terrible taste in the mouth, retreating gums, framing of profound pockets between teeth and gums, detached or moving teeth, changes in the way teeth fit together after chomping down, or in the fit of fractional dentures. Regardless of the possibility that you don't recognize any manifestations, you may even now have some level of gum sickness. In some individuals, gum malady may influence just certain teeth, for example, the molars.

Just a dental specialist or a periodontist can perceive and focus the movement of gum illness.

How Does My Dental Practitioner Diagnose Gum Illness?

Throughout a dental exam, your dental practitioner normally checks for these things: Gum dying, swelling, immovability, and pocket profundity (the space between the gum and tooth; the bigger and deeper the pocket, the more extreme the ailment); development and legitimate teeth arrangement; your jawbone, to help discover the breakdown of bone encompassing your teeth.

How is Gum Sickness Treated?

The objectives of gum sickness medicine are to push reattachment of solid gums to teeth; diminish swelling, the profundity of pockets, and the danger of disease; and to stop infection movement. Medication choices rely upon the phase of malady, how you may have reacted to prior medicines, and your general well-being. Choices range from non-surgical helps that control bacterial development to surgery to restore steady tissues. A full portrayal of the different medication alternatives is given in Gum Disease Treatments.

Ways to Prevent Gum Diseases

Gum illness could be turned around in about all situations when fitting plaque control is drilled. Legitimate plaque control comprises of expert cleaning twice a year and daily brushing and flossing. Brushing dispenses with plaque from the surfaces of the teeth; flossing expels sustenance particles and plaque from in the middle of the teeth and under the gum line. Antibacterial mouth flushes can decrease microbes that cause plaque and gum ailment, as per the American Dental Association.

How Can Gum Infection be Counteracted? proceeded...

Other well-being and lifestyle changes that will diminish the danger, seriousness, and pace of gum ailment progression include:

Stop smoking. Tobacco utilization is a noteworthy danger element for progression of periodontitis. Smokers are seven times more likely to get gum ailment than non-smokers, and smoking can bring down the shots of accomplishment of a few medicines.

Decrease stress. Anxiety may make it troublesome for your body's resistant framework to battle off disease. Keep up a decently adjusted eating methodology. Legitimate sustenance helps your immune system battle disease. Consuming nourishments with cancer prevention agent properties - for instance, those holding vitamin E (vegetable oils, nuts, green verdant vegetables) and vitamin C (citrus foods grown from the ground, broccoli, potatoes) - can help your body repair harmed tissue.

The Overall Health Benefits Beyond Oral Care

Ancient Ayurvedic well-being experts accepted that oil pulling could decrease more than simple ailments of the mouth and throat. Today, numerous encompassing experts tout the utilization of oil for an assortment of well-being concerns.

It is believed that these oils help the lymphatic arrangement of the body by evacuating unsafe microscopic organisms and valuable micro verdure which are given a solid environment to thrive. Because of this comprehensive viewpoint, oil pulling has been utilized as a protective well-being measure for many different conditions.

Other possible benefits of oil pulling for overall health include:

- Detoxification of the body from harmful metals and organisms.

- Reduces the symptoms of allergy.

- Aids in reducing pain.

- Prevent heart disease.

- Improve your skin.

- Reduce hangover after alcohol consumption.

- Helps reduce insomnia.

- Some people report improved vision.

- May help in reducing sinus congestion.

- Help support normal kidney function.

- May reduce symptoms of bronchitis.

- Aids in the reduction of eczema.

- May help with gastroenteritis.

- Reducing inflammation of arthritis.

- Correcting hormonal imbalances.

- Migraine headache relief.

Conclusion

There are various ways of keeping ourselves healthy and away from diseases, such as maintaining proper hygiene. Although oil pulling is also believed by some to be effective in health maintenance and healthy living, it is not wise to rely solely on it. Always remember that there is no diverse scientific research that has been performed to certify the claims of oil pulling. To be on the safe side, it is usually better to have a routine check up at the hospital. If you otherwise choose also to embrace the qualities of oil pulling, then it should be done in such a manner that care holds the upper hand.